My Four Secrets

FOR A SUCCESSFUL IVF CYCLE

DR. MARYAM MAHANIAN, DTCM, RAc
Doctor of Traditional Chinese Medicine & Registered Acupuncturist

My Four Secrets for a Successful IVF Cycle

Copyright © 2020 Dr. Maryam Mahanian

All rights reserved.

ISBN: 9798648956490

Dedication

This guide is dedicated to all the couples struggling with the heartbreak of infertility

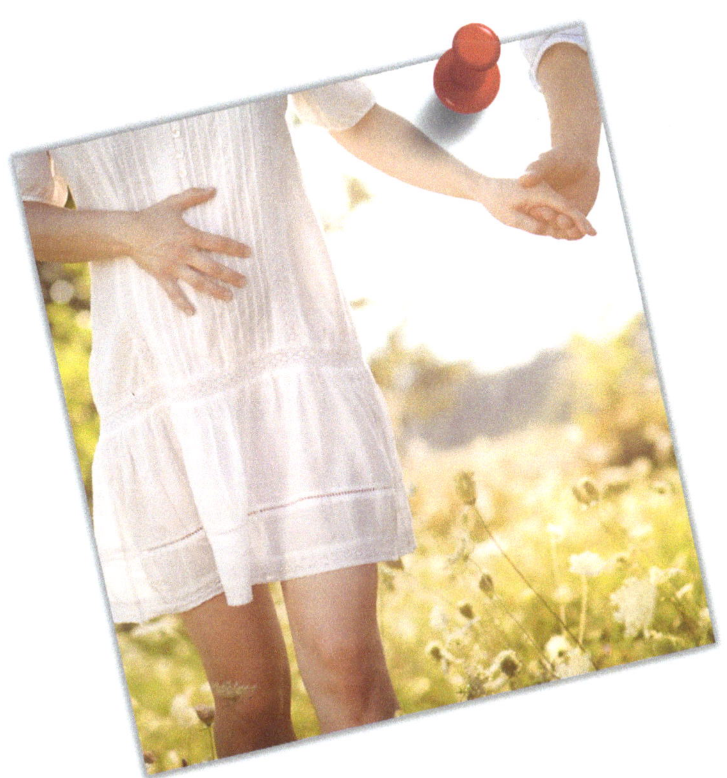

Contents

Introduction

BECOMING A MOM!

Can you imagine what it would feel like to become a mom and hold your miracle baby in your arms?

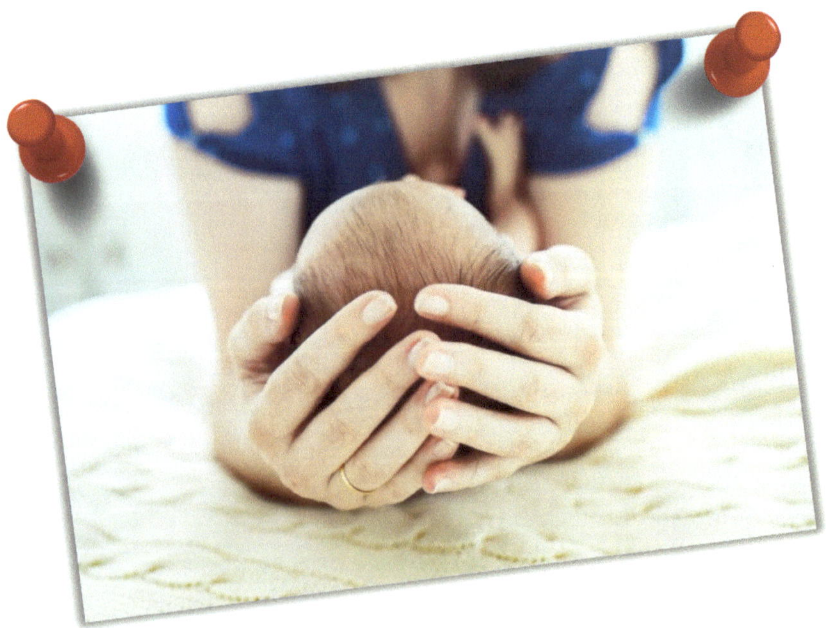

My goal is to educate you on how you can improve your chances of becoming pregnant with your IVF cycle so that holding your baby will become a reality.

WHY I WROTE THIS GUIDE

Since starting my Chinese medical practice in 2002, I've treated many couples who sought out Chinese medicine because they wanted to start a family. The number of people who have some degree of infertility now is one in four couples. To me, these numbers are alarming and tell me that there is such a need to help these couples grow the families they have always dreamed of having.

Of the couples that are dealing with fertility issues, many of them seek out alternative therapies like Traditional Chinese medicine. This includes modalities such as acupuncture, acupressure, Chinese food cures and Chinese herbal medicine.

The reason so many couples are attracted to Chinese medicine is because Chinese medicine works! It's a wonderful supportive therapy when you're doing IVF. It's also a good stand-alone therapy to improve fertility if you're not going through the IVF process.

The reason why I wrote this guide is because I've gotten the question time and time again "what can I do to increase the chance of my IVF working"? While my online course, IVF With Confidence, teaches you the exact things you can do at home while undergoing an IVF cycle, this guide has a different purpose.

This guide speaks mostly about Chinese medicine and not of the particulars of the IVF stages and processes.

This guide demystifies and explains the advantages and benefits of Chinese medicine used in combination with IVF. This guide is also advantageous for those trying to get pregnant naturally.

My hope is that this information will give you some insight into the wisdom of Chinese medicine and its role in improving IVF success to get you pregnant.

You have probably heard of Chinese medicine and acupuncture before. Perhaps you know someone who swears by it. You may have a friend who has tried it to improve their fertility, or regulate their cycle, balance their hormones or reduce their stress. But you may not understand how it works and what it entails. The purpose of this guide is to give you a better understanding of how Traditional Chinese medicine can support you in your IVF process.

IVF IS NOT A GUARANTEE

The reality is that IVF can be an emotional, physical and financial roller coaster ride! While success rates are climbing slightly due to better techniques being used and more technology in IVF clinics, **it's still not a guarantee that you'll get pregnant with IVF**.

The odds of success with IVF are between **34% and 42%** for women of all ages over three IVF cycles. So let's do everything we can to put you in the success category!

Number of Couples Seeking Complementary Medicine is Steadily on the Rise

Two out of three couples choose complementary medicine like Chinese medicine alongside Western medicine treatments like IVF in the US. In Europe this rate is much higher.

> *I strongly urge you to seek Chinese medicine if you haven't already. The aim of this guide is to help you better understand Chinese medicine, how it can support your IVF cycle and inspire you to become proactive in your fertility journey.*

Chapter

1

CHAPTER ONE: WHAT YOU NEED FOR A SUCCESSFUL IVF CYCLE

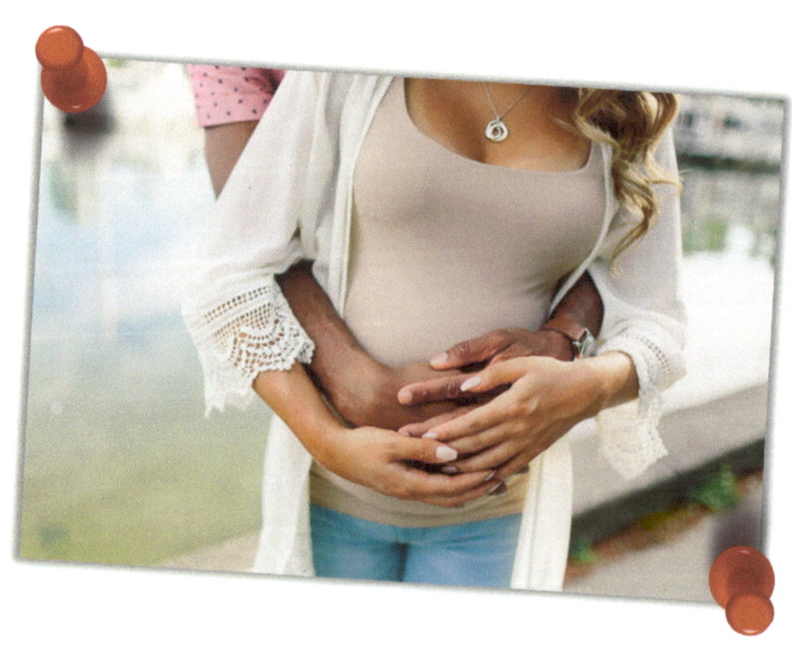

From the standpoint of Traditional Chinese Medicine, there are a number of prerequisites that need to be in place to maximize the rate of success of an IVF cycle. In Jane Lyttleton's textbook "The Treatment of Infertility with Chinese Medicine", she includes the following:

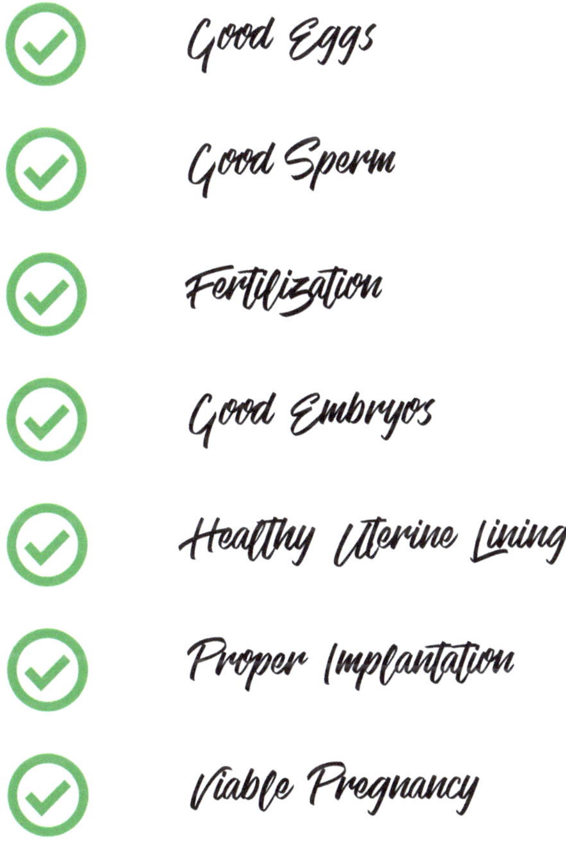

GOOD EGGS

This (with good sperm) is the most important stage.

Chinese medicine can enhance egg and sperm quality. Western fertility drugs increase the quantity of eggs but actually can't do very much for the quality of the eggs.

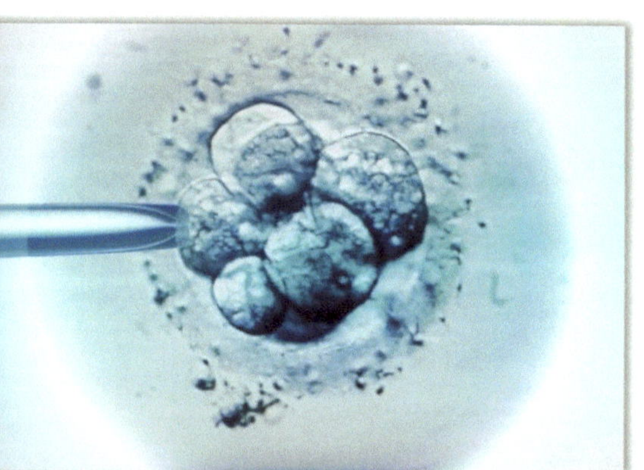

Improve the quality of eggs for 3 months (or 90 days) prior to your IVF cycle. It takes three months for follicles to develop and mature before the egg is ovulated and the environment of the follicle at that time is key for good egg quality.

GOOD SPERM

It takes approximately seventy-four days for sperm to mature so typically it takes this long for a man who is making improvements in his health to start to see changes in his sperm quality. In the clinic setting, I round up this number and tell my male patients to try for at least three months of treatment prior to their IVF cycles.

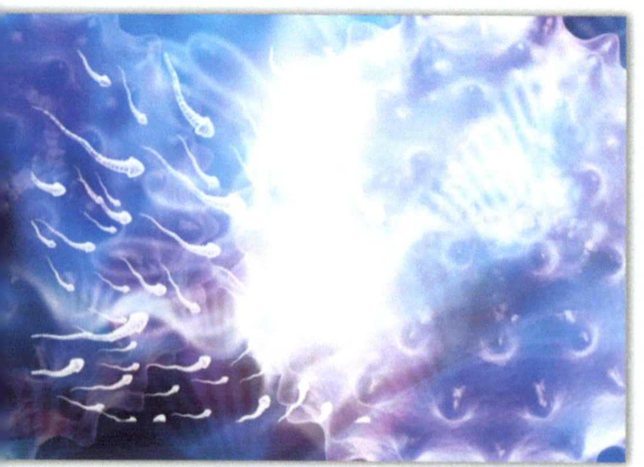

FERTILIZATION

This is what IVF is particularly great at! If one has blocked fallopian tubes or the sperm is unable to reach the egg for a variety of reasons, IVF creates a brilliant solution.

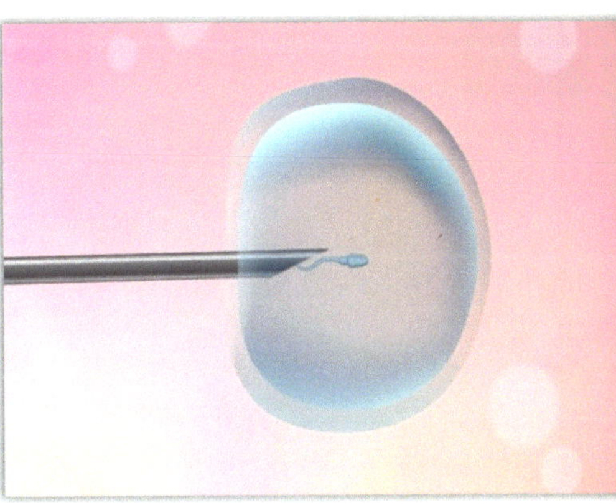

ICDI or IntraCytoplasmic Sperm Injection is also an option for couples where sperm are unable to fertilize the egg. For example, ICDI might be implemented if there is low sperm count, low sperm motility (movement) or morphology (shape), or if there is any physical blockages preventing the sperm from fertilizing the egg. ICSI is a specialized technique used in IVF where a single sperm cell is injected into the cytoplasm of the egg.

GOOD EMBRYOS

Both Chinese medicine and IVF are of great help at this stage. Good embryos are a function of three things:

- the quality of both the sperm and the egg
- how well the sperm and the egg fuse together
- the compatibility of the sperm and egg's genetic material

Chinese medicine will help the sperm and the egg quality.

IVF will help with the sperm and the egg getting together and the egg becoming fertilized. Therefore, **both Chinese medicine and IVF are very important for good quality embryos**.

HEALTHY UTERINE LINING

A good uterine lining will predict good embryo implantation.

If your uterine lining is too thin, this has been shown to cause

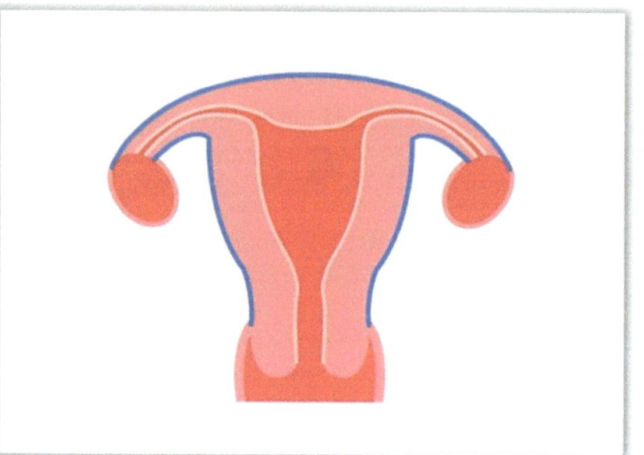

unexplained IVF failure or recurrent miscarriage.

Chinese medicine will improve the thickness and the quality of the lining. It does this, in a nutshell, by improving blood flow to the uterus and increasing progesterone levels.

PROPER IMPLANTATION

Implantation will occur if the embryo is strong and the development of the uterine lining is appropriate.

As said earlier, Chinese medicine improves blood flow to the uterus to support proper implantation. In IVF, aspirin is often given which also encourages blood flow.

VIABLE PREGNANCY

This will depend on all the previous factors leading up to this phase. If those steps have been successful, then it is very likely the pregnancy will lead to a healthy baby. Chinese medicine can greatly help in the first trimester of pregnancy to reduce the chances of a miscarriage to occur.

Summary of how Chinese medicine contributes to a successful IVF cycle to get pregnant:

- Helps ovaries respond better to the stimulation drugs used in IVF
- Balances hormones
- Improves egg quality
- Improves sperm quality
- Relieves the side effects of fertility drugs
- Improves the thickness and quality of the uterine lining
- Helps implantation

Can you imagine how much you would benefit from supercharging your IVF procedure by enhancing its effectiveness by as much as 50%, while at the same time reducing its side effects on your body?

Of course, nobody wants an unsuccessful IVF cycle. The process is hard enough physically and mentally, not to mention failed attempts or the mental trauma of a miscarriage. It can be very hard on relationships.

I want you to imagine what life could be like to get through IVF for the last time, and have that miracle baby, while feeling your best both mentally and physically.

So if you're already mentally ready to undergo IVF, you're already in the right mindset to give it your best shot, and Chinese medicine can be the catalyst to help you get there and see better results.

THE TOOLS, TIPS AND TRICKS

Chinese medicine gives you the guidance, tools, and all the tips you need every step of the way at each phase of your IVF cycle for you to get the most out of your IVF cycle while also improving your health. **This is backed by science.**

The one thing that I really want you to understand is that there are things you can do to improve the success of your IVF cycle and get pregnant.

> *You can go from feeling overwhelmed, uncertain and intimidated by your IVF process to feeling confident that you're doing everything you can to make the most out of your IVF cycle and finally get pregnant.*

Okay, So Let's Get To The Good Stuff.

In this handbook, I've narrowed down the four most important secrets (or ingredients) to having success with IVF. These are what I have found to be **the most effective and most important for my patients to get pregnant with IVF** over the last two decades.

Chapter

2

CHAPTER TWO: THE ADVANTAGES OF TRADITIONAL CHINESE MEDICINE

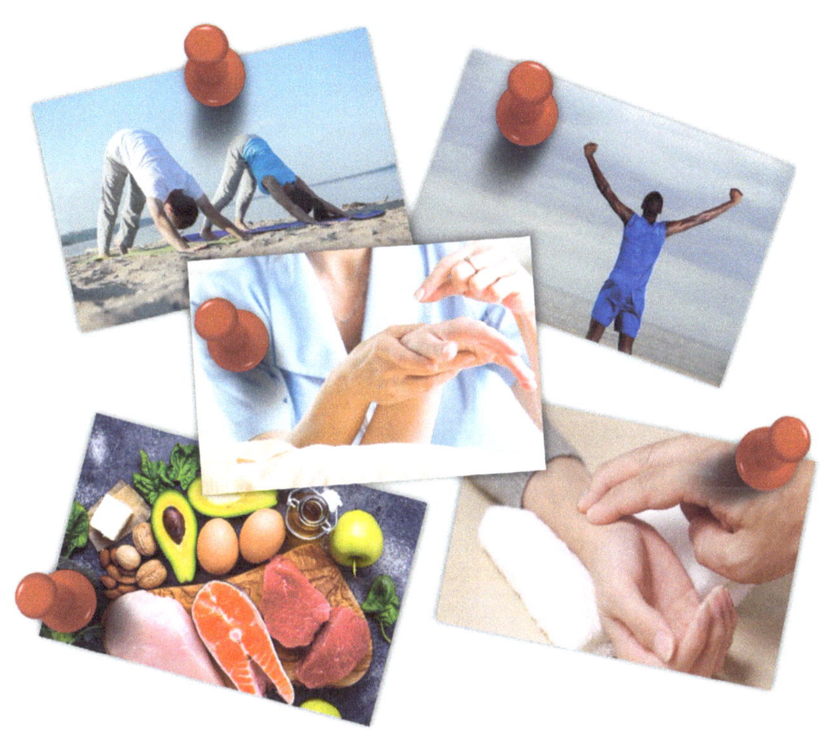

CHINESE MEDICINE IS SAFE

It goes without saying that not all "natural" remedies or practices are safe. Natural practices can be very powerful and have dramatic influences on our bodies. This is where a qualified practitioner guiding you along this journey is so important.

When you have guidance from a qualified practitioner of Chinese medicine, Chinese medicine treatments are safe and have minimal or no side effects.

When it comes to acupuncture or acupressure though, I can quite safely say that the risk of experiencing any side effects is extremely low.

There is a growing body of solid evidence that states that acupuncture and Chinese medicine are safe and effective for many situations, including and not limited to fertility and IVF support. You have nothing to lose when you implement Chinese medicine solutions and so much to gain.

CHINESE MEDICINE IS EVIDENCE-BASED

Of all the different complementary and alternative medicine

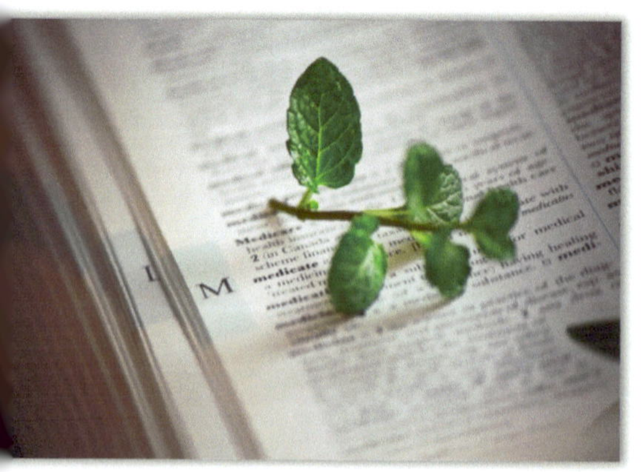

therapies, Traditional Chinese medicine had undergone the most testing and research.

Although most of the research has been conducted on acupuncture and Chinese herbal medicine, there has also been extensive research done on other modalities of

TCM including moxibustion, acupressure, cupping and Qigong.

Chinese medicine practitioners are hoping for more "whole system TCM" research rather than research that has been focused on one specific modality like acupuncture or Chinese herbal medicine. Whole system TCM includes acupuncture, acupressure, diet and nutrition and lifestyle changes.

For IVF support, "whole system TCM" has greater odds of live birth compared to IVF alone or IVF with acupuncture administered only on the day of embryo transfer. Source: National Center for Biotechnology Information Search database: https://www.ncbi.nlm.nih.gov/pmc/articles/PMC4458185/

For example, in my online self-treatment course, IVF With Confidence, I take more of a whole systems approach where I teach various Chinese medicine techniques and tools that support the IVF cycle and improve overall health from home

CHINESE MEDICINE IS CUSTOMIZED

Because Chinese medicine is customized specifically to the individual, that's what makes it so effective. People have different constitutions. This means every individual has a different body type that makes them unique but can change over time. The health of your body's constitution depends on your diet, lifestyle, and genetics. It even goes back to the health of your parents at the time you were conceived.

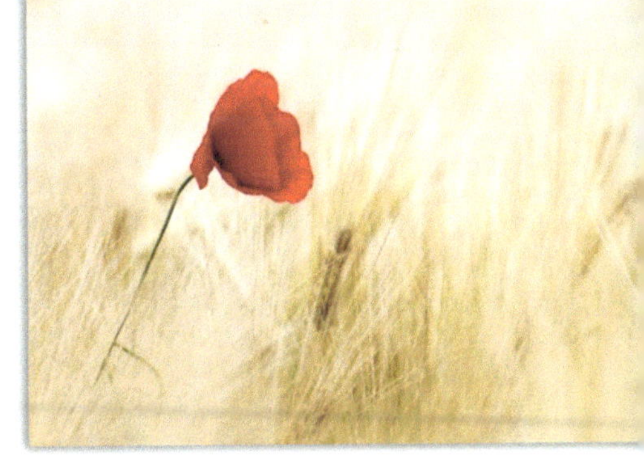

When you see a practitioner of Chinese medicine, after doing a thorough health assessment with you, they will give you a constitutional diagnosis. You may be too damp; you may have Qi deficiency, yang deficiency, yin deficiency, Qi stagnation and so

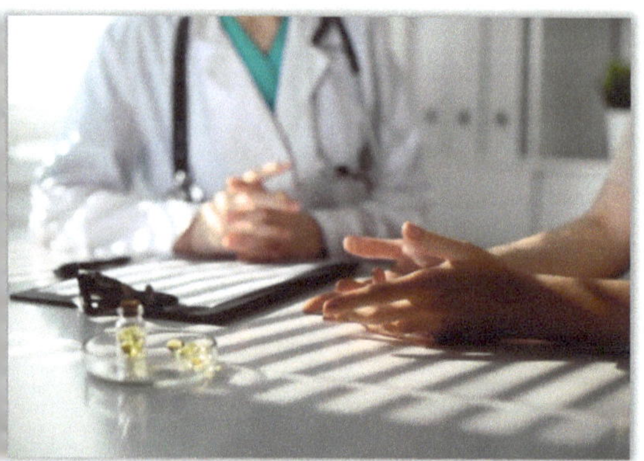

forth. The treatment protocol that you receive will depend on your constitutional diagnosis. Sometimes even the small tweaks in your lifestyle will create balance in your body and better health.

CHINESE MEDICINE IS TIME-TESTED DATING BACK THOUSANDS OF YEARS

Who can argue with a medicine that has been around for thousands of years and continues to be used by millions of people? Chinese

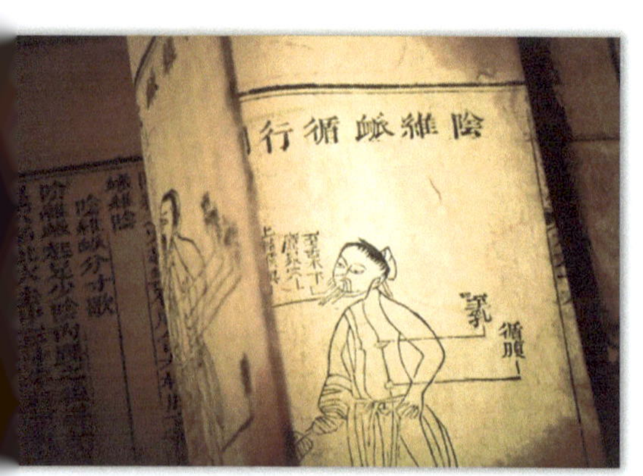

medicine treatment for women's health is no exception to this. There are Chinese classics that date back thousands of years that talk about the anatomy, physiology, diagnosis and treatment of women's diseases.

CHINESE MEDICINE CAN TREAT A WIDE RANGE OF CONDITIONS

In this guide we're of course focusing on IVF support, but I can't help but mention here that Chinese medicine has the ability to treat a very wide range of conditions. Everything from skin issues, hormonal imbalances, pain, digestive problems, infections, allergies and colds and flus to name a few. Chinese medicine is even being widely used to enhance beauty and anti-aging.

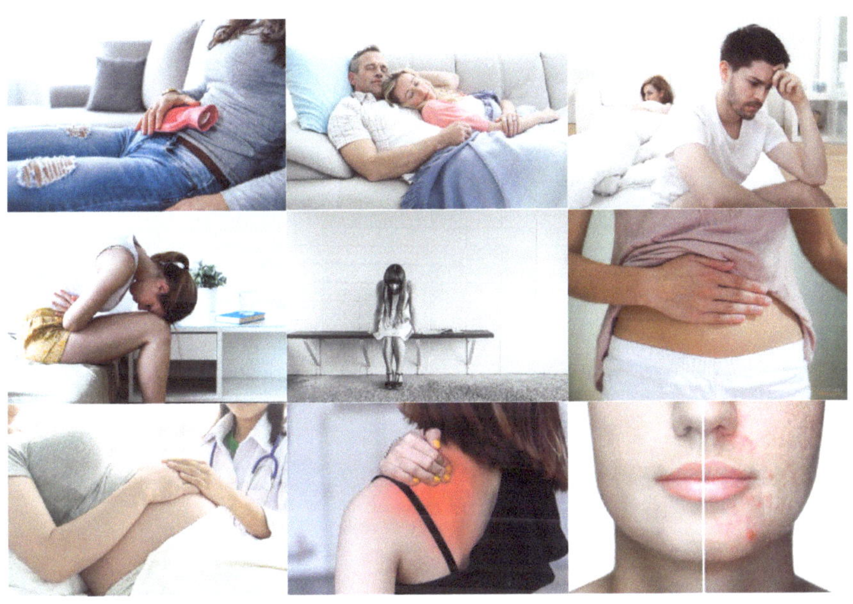

CHINESE MEDICINE SHINES IN THE AREA OF WOMEN'S HEALTH, FERTILITY & IVF SUPPORT

Chinese medicine excels at adjusting imbalances to improve fertility and women's health issues. This is why you've probably seen many acupuncture clinics specialized in fertility. Their entire practices are focused on it. Why? Because it works so well!

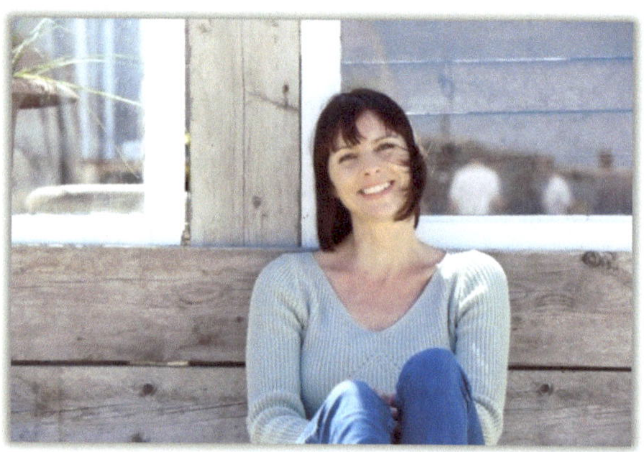

BENEFITS YOUR FERTILITY & YOUR OVERALL WELL-BEING

While your main goal is to improve your fertility and have your miracle baby, getting Chinese medicine treatment will also benefit your overall health and well-being - It can boost your immune system and energy, improve your emotional well-being, fight depression and calm anxiety.

CHINESE HERBAL MEDICINE DOES NOT ADD HORMONES

The common treatment for hormonal imbalance in the way of deficiency of hormones is in the form of the birth control pill, hormone replacement therapy and bioidentical hormones. Chinese medicine is a bit different. It aims to facilitate your body's endocrine system to balance and adjust by itself with the end result being hormone regulation. It allows for your body to produce its own hormones and to also respond better to the endocrine system. It does this in a subtle and delicate way.

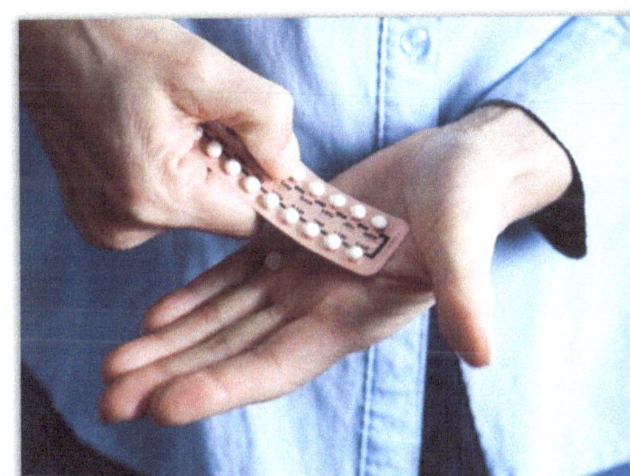

TCM TREATS THE ROOT CAUSE

Another wonderful aspect of Chinese medicine is that it offers a permanent solution. It can treat the root cause. When a certain imbalance is corrected, and the individual keeps up their part to play in maintaining a good diet and lifestyle, the harmony in the body continues.

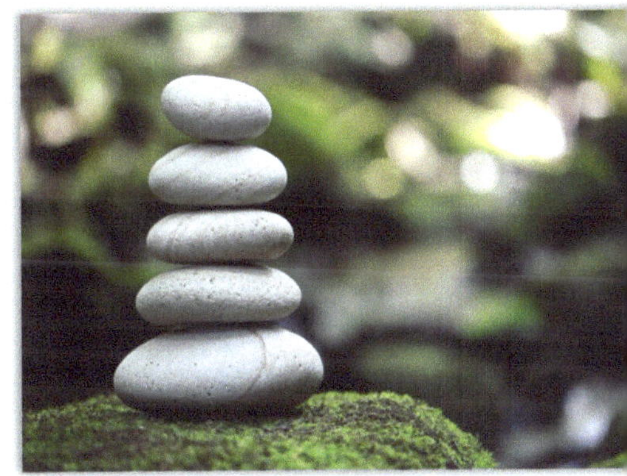

TAKES MIND, BODY, SPIRIT AND EMOTIONAL WELL-BEING INTO ACCOUNT ALL AT THE SAME TIME

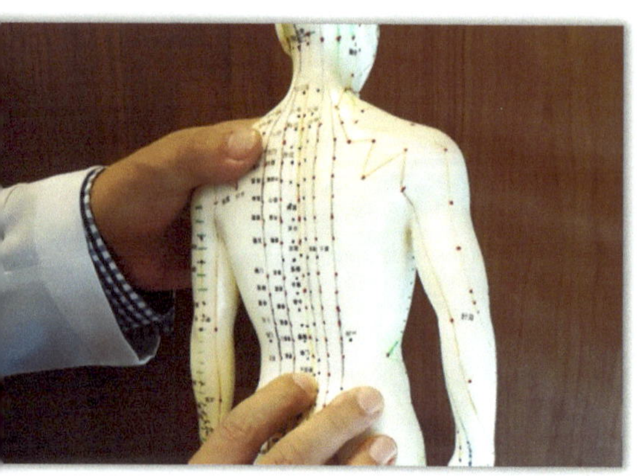

We know that the mind, body, spirit and emotions are tightly interconnected and can't be separated. Chinese medicine will treat all of the above simultaneously.

CHINESE MEDICINE IS RELATIVELY LOW-COST COMPARED TO FERTILITY TREATMENTS LIKE IVF

While the cost of Chinese medicine and acupuncture can definitely add up over time, it is still a much less expensive process than fertility treatments like IVF.

Chapter

3

CHAPTER THREE: FOUNDATIONS OF CHINESE MEDICINE & FERTILITY

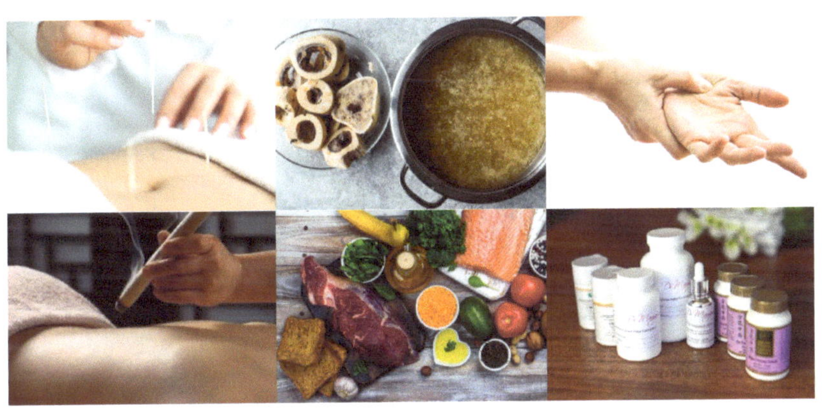

It's important to give you some basic foundational information on Chinese medicine before moving on too much further in this guide.

TOOLS/MODALITIES USED IN CHINESE MEDICINE:

Acupuncture, acupressure, Chinese herbal medicine, diet and nutrition, Moxibustion are all important tools that help support a successful IVF Cycle. And while the step-by-step application of these tools and modalities are taught in my online IVF course "IVF With Confidence" it would be impossible to capture this information in its entirely within the scope of this guide. Instead, a cursory review of these tools and modalities are provided in this guide.

YIN AND YANG

This is a central concept in Chinese medicine. Yin and yang are opposite forces in nature. Everything in our world has its yin and yang aspects. Yin is inward energy, female, night, cooling, stillness, fluids, substance. Yang is outward energy, male, daytime, warming

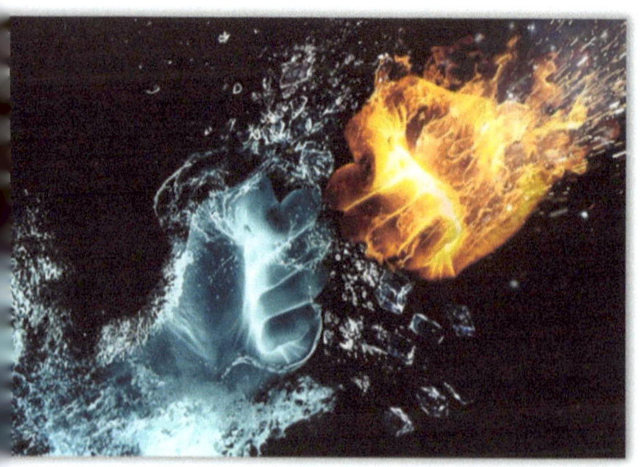

and activity. In order to be healthy, there needs to be a delicate balance between yin and yang within our bodies. This is especially apparent when it comes to improving our fertility.

QI (PRONOUNCED "CHEE")

Qi is very loosely translated as "energy" or "life force". Qi moves through our bodies through meridians or channels. Qi and blood move together as Qi is actually the force that moves the blood with it and blood carries the Qi along with it.

When it comes to our health, we need proper flow of Qi and we need adequate amounts of it. Otherwise we will have Qi blockage or Qi deficiency. This can negatively impact fertility and the success of your IVF cycle.

BLOOD

Blood is nourishment. It is what sustains the body.

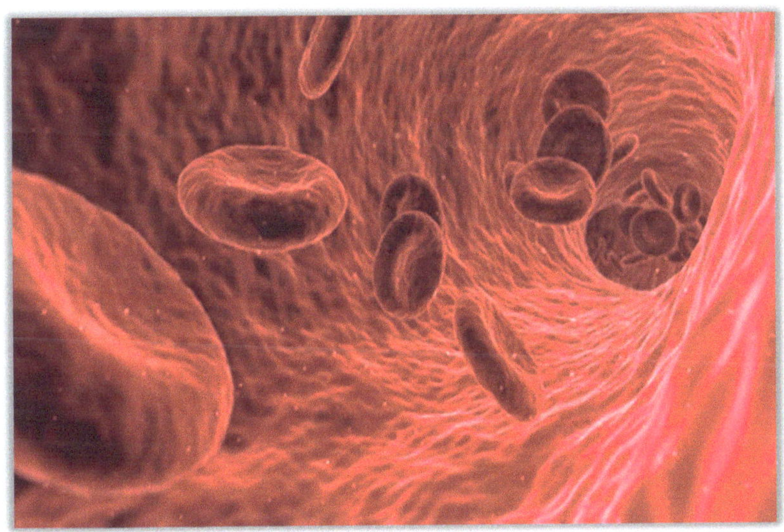

Blood is responsible for providing nutrients, oxygen and moisture to the organs, tissues, bones, muscles and channels (meridians).

Qi and blood have an extremely close association. Similar to the close association that yin and yang have.

OPTIMAL HEALTH

When it comes to our health, any excess, deficiency or stagnation of Qi, blood, yin and yang can lead to imbalance and will cause a disruption in optimal health. Optimal health means balance or equilibrium. It's when the body is in a state of homeostasis.

KIDNEY-ESSENCE (JING)

There are different types of kidney-essence (another word for essence is Jing) but we won't get into them in great detail in this guide. Kidney-essence provides the most basic material that makes up the organs and tissues and maintains the life activities of the human body. Kidney-essence is the foundation for both kidney-yin and kidney-yang.

Essence belongs to yin (substance) and Qi belongs to yang (function).

KIDNEY-ESSENCE AND REPRODUCTION

Kidney-essence is responsible for growth, development, sexual maturity, reproduction and pregnancy in Chinese medicine. Kidney-essence is the basis of conception.

We will get into more specifics about the kidney organ system and how it pertains to fertility later in this chapter.

MERIDIANS (AKA: CHANNELS) & NETWORK VESSELS

The meridians in our bodies each connect with a specific organ system. It is these meridians and their network vessels that connect the organ systems with one another. The vital substances already discussed such as qi, blood and body fluids all run throughout these channels.

These meridians are similar to a highway system that runs throughout the entire body. It's a vast and complicated system that takes years to study and understand. For the purposes of this guide for IVF support, all I want you to understand about these channels is that proper movement of Qi, blood and body fluids within these channels is key. Otherwise, you'll have disruption in proper flow and lack of proper nourishment to the organ systems.

OPTIMAL FERTILITY NEEDS A BALANCE OF YIN, YANG, QI, BLOOD AND ESSENCE

When any of these factors is out of balance, it makes proper fertility that much harder. The delicate balance of the hormones, organs and energy systems is what leads to a healthy conception, pregnancy and best of all a healthy baby.

THE THREE MAIN ORGAN SYSTEMS

In Chinese medicine, there are three main organ systems involved in reproduction. These include the **Kidneys**, **Liver**, and **Spleen**.

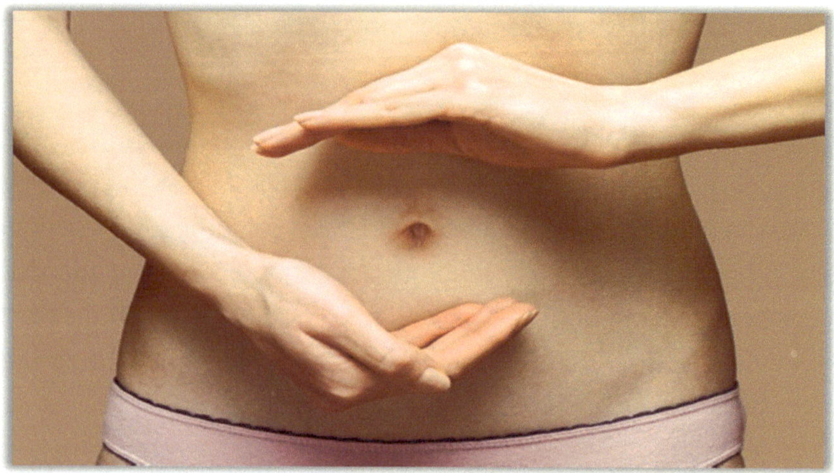

THE KIDNEYS

We have touched on the kidneys already but let's dig a little deeper.

- The kidneys control the endocrine & reproductive systems
- The kidneys are responsible for our genetics
- The kidneys are in charge of growth and development.
- The kidneys store essence and essence is the material basis of the menstrual blood. The kidney essence has a great influence on puberty, fertility, conception, pregnancy and menopause. Aging depletes essence.

THE LIVER

The liver organ system is vital when it comes to fertility. It has an important connection to the uterus and the blood. Here are a few reasons:

Liver stores the blood

The liver is often called the "woman's organ". As said above, it has a relationship with the uterus and the blood. The liver stores the blood so the uterus depends on the liver to receive the blood. Therefore, the liver system is directly involved with menstruation.

Liver moves the Qi

The liver organ system is the primary organ that ensures our menstrual cycles are regular. It is the liver-Qi that moves the blood in order for the menstrual period to occur. If there is blockage of the liver Qi, it may cause irregular periods, PMS or menstrual cramps.

The liver calms emotional energy

The liver becomes blocked or congested when we are stressed, anxious, frustrated, tense, angry and have unfulfilled desires. We have all heard of the negative impact that stress can have on fertility. The liver congestion that results with this stress impedes the proper flow of Qi and blood.

THE SPLEEN

The Spleen produces Qi and blood

The spleen is very important to fertility, particularly female fertility since females are more prone to having a deficiency of blood.

The spleen produces blood and Qi and this blood is then stored in the liver.

In Chinese medicine, the spleen and stomach are in charge of our digestion. The food and drinks that we ingest are broken down in the stomach and it's the function of the spleen to transform and transport those nutrients to make Qi and blood.

Spleen holds the Qi

Another aspect of the spleen with its relation to fertility & pregnancy is the fact that the spleen holds the Qi. The spleen keeps the uterus in place. Sinking of spleen Qi can cause uterus prolapse.

The Spleen holds the blood in the vessels

The spleen also "contains the blood". If the spleen is weak, blood will leak out of its vessels causing bleeding and heavy periods.

Chapter

4

CHAPTER FOUR: SECRET NO.1 - BLOOD FLOW

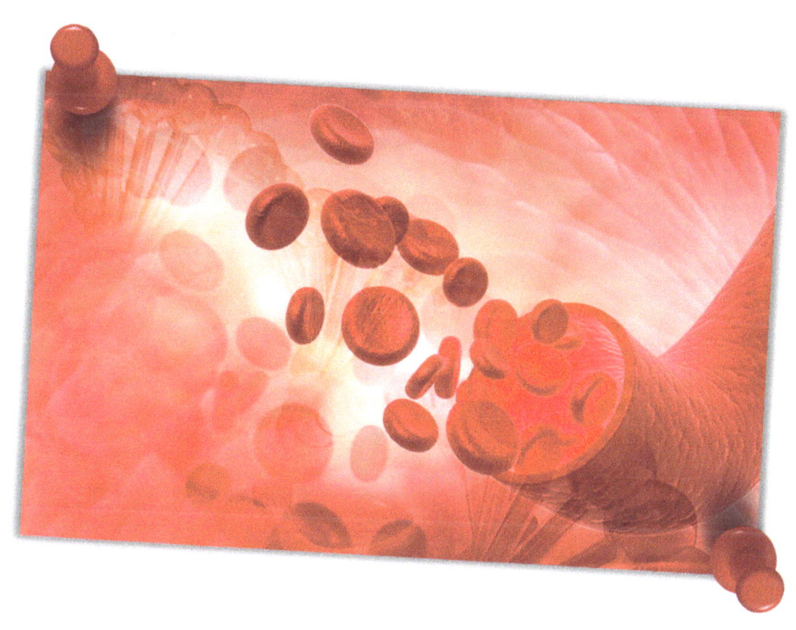

Now for the exciting stuff. My **first secret** to improve your IVF success: **Blood Flow**.

In Chinese medicine, blood flow is everything! Activating adequate blood circulation is the treatment method for many different conditions but is especially important when it comes to fertility and your IVF success.

HORMONES, OXYGEN, NUTRIENTS AND MOISTURE

Better blood flow to the ovaries and uterus means with more blood comes more hormones, oxygen, nutrients and moisture.

This will allow for a better environment when the follicles are maturing and growing. This also helps hormone balance and helps ovaries respond better to the stimulation fertility drugs involved in the IVF process.

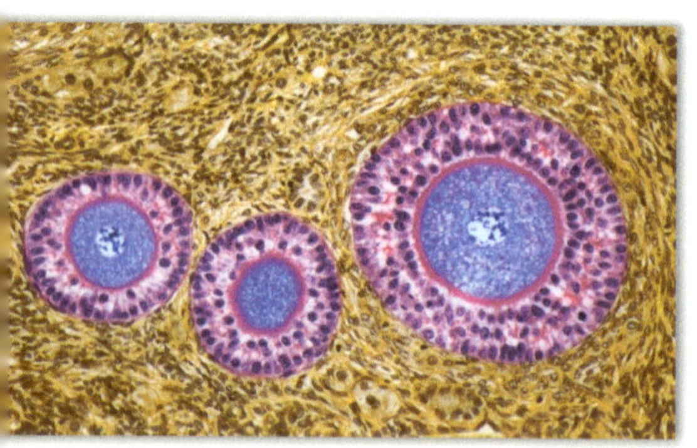

Colour-Doppler Studies have shown that follicular development is directly related to their blood supply. Good quality blood supply to the follicle during ovarian stimulation has been associated with a greater likelihood of recovering a mature egg, higher grade embryos and an improved chance of healthy pregnancy.

Unfortunately, poor blood supply can result in a longer stimulation phase being required and fewer eggs being recruited.

Healthy circulation promotes healing and helps to break down scar tissue and adhesions.

Better blood flow also helps to promote ovulation.

Proper blood flow is vital to a good quality thick uterine lining. **Better blood flow = better uterine lining**. A thick receptive nourishing uterine lining is the best possible environment for the embryo to thrive.

A good uterine lining is at least 7 to 8mm thick and displays a trilaminar (3 layered) appearance on ultrasound.

A trilaminar appearance: These are three lines in your uterine lining. The thickness of the uterine lining is the distance between two external lines.

Your uterine lining gets thicker in response to hormones. It's the action of estrogen, in the first half of your menstrual cycle (the follicular phase) leading up to ovulation that stimulates the uterine lining to thicken and create a trilaminar (three layered) appearance.

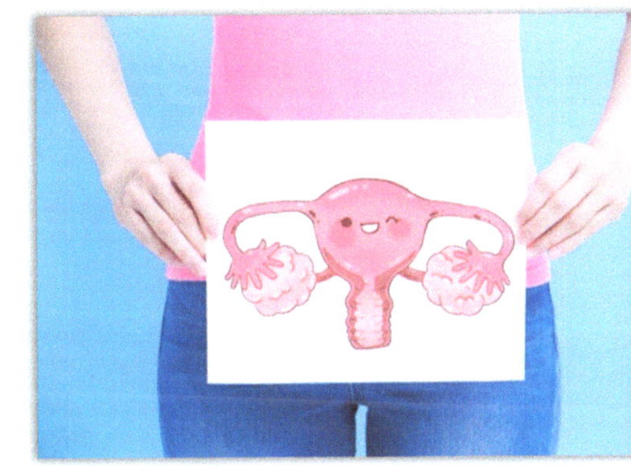

Having a thin uterine lining doesn't entirely mean that you won't get pregnant but it does mean that implantation may be more difficult. Doctors call the "window of implantation" the period of time that the uterus is in its best state for implantation to happen. If your uterine lining is too thin, it will negatively affect your window of implantation.

A lining that is too thin can lead to failed implantation or early pregnancy loss.

There was a research study published in *Fertility and Sterility* where they found that acupuncture reduced constriction in the uterine arteries which increases the blood flow to the ovaries and uterus. This can dramatically increase the success of IVF. It was found that acupuncture reduces the sympathetic fight or flight response in stressful situations. When this sympathetic response is reduced, blood flow to the reproductive organs increases. https://www.ncbi.nlm.nih.gov/pubmed/8671446

FUNCTIONS OF THE BLOOD

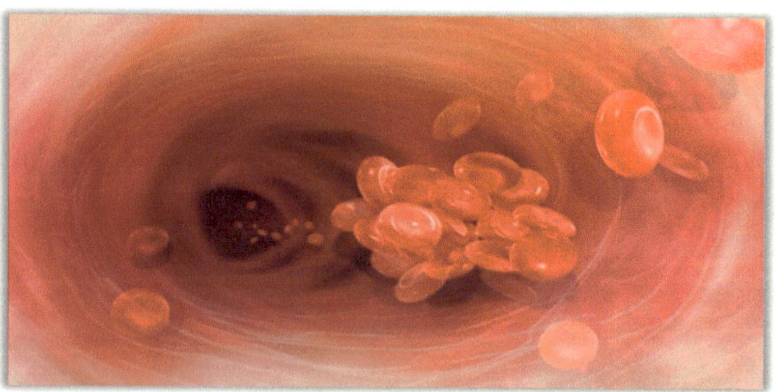

Here are some of the many great functions of the blood according to Western medicine:

- The blood takes the nutrients from the digestion to all body parts including the organs, tissues, skin etc.
- The blood transports hormones from the endocrine system to target areas
- The blood carries waste out to the lungs
- The blood transports oxygen from the lungs to all parts of the body including the reproductive organs
- The blood circulates heat throughout the body
- The blood removes toxins and wastes from the body

How does Chinese medicine improve the flow of blood?

- By nourishing blood so that there is more of it to flow within the vessels. Blood deficiency leads to blood stagnation.
- By relieving stuck blood and stuck Qi
- By adding warmth to move the blood. Warmth is needed as a catalyst to move blood. The opposite is true of cold which impedes the flow of blood.

Some examples of blood deficiency signs and symptoms

- light period flow or no periods;
- delayed periods;
- dry symptoms such as dry skin, dry hair, dry eyes, dry mouth;
- hair loss or thinning hair;
- pale complexion, dizziness, blurry vision, insomnia

Some examples of blood stagnation signs and symptoms

- Menstrual cramps;
- clots in the menstrual blood;
- dark menstrual blood;
- delayed or irregular periods;
- pain in the body;
- dark complexion;
- abdominal masses like cysts or myomas

Blood cold

- all the same symptoms as blood stagnation (i.e. menstrual cramps, clots in the menstrual blood, dark menstrual blood, delayed or irregular periods, generalized pain in the body, dark complexion and/or masses) with the addition of cold signs like cold body, hands and feet and pale complexion.

There are different ways of improving blood flow to the reproductive organs to give you the best chances of IVF success. In fact, there are techniques that can be applied at home to achieve this and I have successfully taught this to my patients thru my online program.

Chapter

5

CHAPTER FIVE: SECRET NO.2 - EGG QUALITY

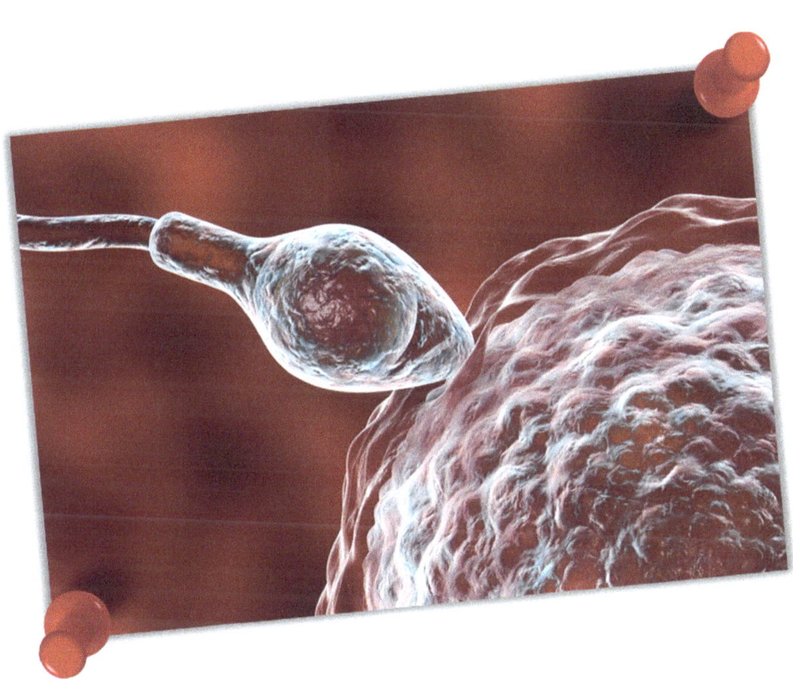

This second secret to success comes as no surprise. Good egg quality. Poor egg quality is one of the most common issues when it comes to infertility.

Good egg quality determines embryo equality

If the egg quality is poor, there may be issues with:

- Implantation
- Chromosomal abnormalities which may lead to miscarriage

Boost energy production by the mitochondria

The concept of improving egg quality is something that many people have heard plenty about and become accustomed to. But there are still many people who are skeptical that there is anything you can do to improve egg quality.

Well, let me take you back to high school Biology for a second. A cell consists of a membrane, a nucleus and cytoplasm. The nucleus is considered the control center where the DNA or genetic material resides. The reason why some are skeptical about the ability to improve egg quality is perhaps because they think that you can't improve an "old" egg or change the genetic material in the nucleus of the egg.

But here is the thing that is important to understand. The cytoplasm of the egg is also important because the mitochondria that produce cellular energy reside in the cytoplasm. It's the mitochondrial energy that contributes to fertilization, the divisions of the embryo and successful implantation. ***By improving on the number and efficiency of the mitochondria, we can actually improve egg quality.***

How do we boost the function of the mitochondria?

- Proper nutrition
- Blood flow
- Oxygen
- Balanced hormones
- Nourish kidney organ system

Let's review some facts about the kidney organ system and kidney-essence:

- it is the basis for reproduction in Chinese medicine
- it has a significant influence on the quality of eggs, sperm and the embryos
- the kidney essence reserves decline with age
- we can consume our kidney Jing by overwork, poor diet, physical and mental strain.
- The good news is that we can replenish the kidney Jing and improve egg quality.

In my Chinese medicine practice, if I suspect poor egg quality to be one of the factors causing infertility in a patient, I ask them if they have certain kidney deficiency signs and symptoms.

Some signs of kidney deficiency are cold hands and feet, low energy, lower back pain, low libido and issues with urination to name a few.

What can negatively affect egg quality?

These are just some of the things that can negatively affect egg quality:

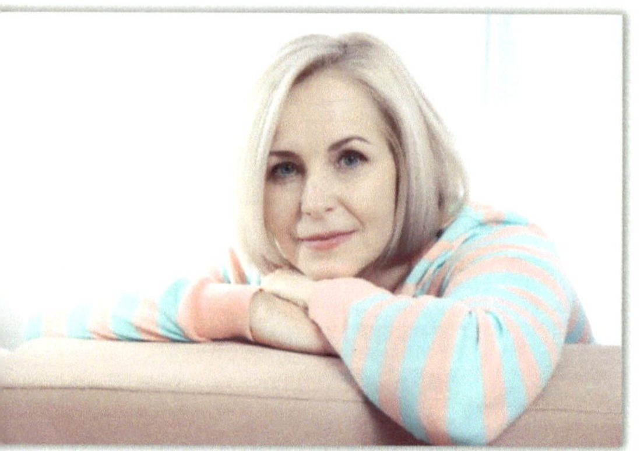

Age: In a younger person's eggs, the mitochondria are more active. In an older person's eggs, like over age 35, the mitochondria are less active and producing less cellular energy.

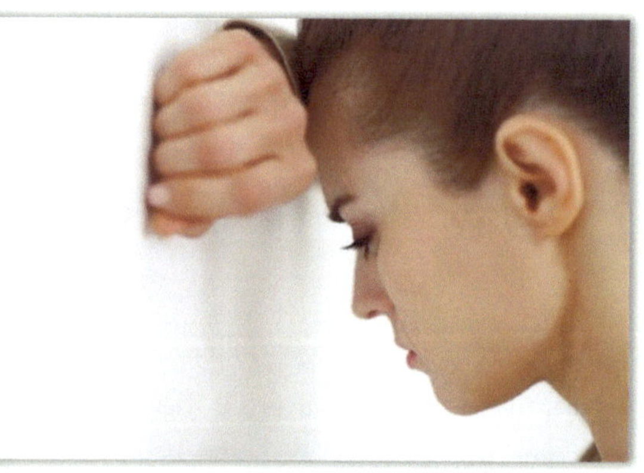

Constant high stress: Stress diverts blood away from the reproductive organs which negatively impacts egg quality. This is because the eggs are in need of the nutrients, hormones, moisture and oxygen that the blood delivers.

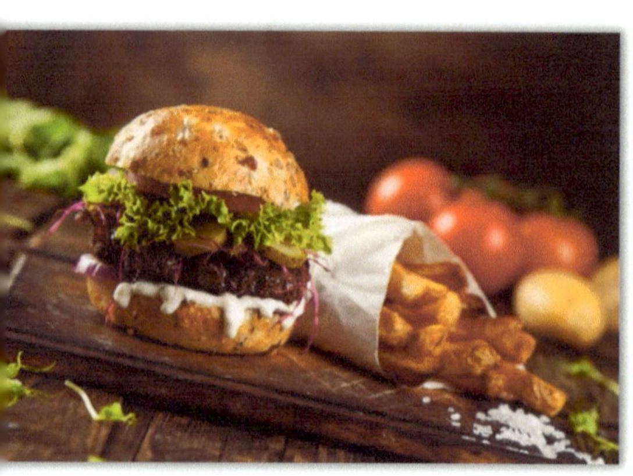

Poor nutrition and being overweight: This can lead to inflammation and hormonal imbalance which can reduce egg quality.

Environmental toxins: These toxins are known as endocrine disruptors which have been shown to cause hormonal imbalances and poor egg quality.

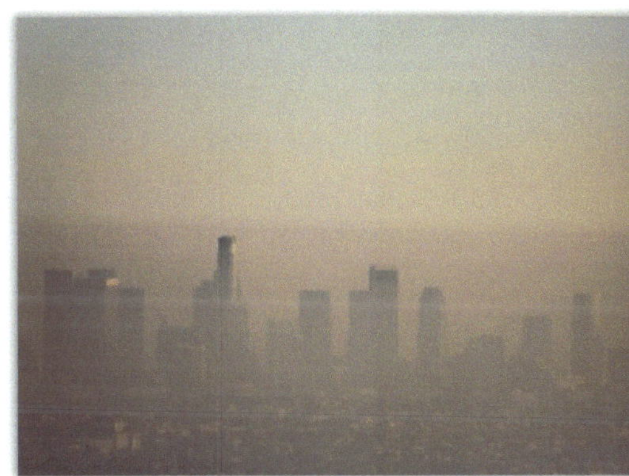

I have successfully taught women thru my online program, IVF With Confidence, how to improve their egg quality for better IVF success. There is **so much you can do at home to improve the environment of the ovaries** to **enable the ovaries to function optimally** and to **support good egg quality**.

100 days

Ideally, if you have time before your IVF cycle, you can take at least 3 months, or 100 days to be exact, to work on egg quality. The reason for this is because **it takes about 100 days for the follicle to mature and develop** before it's released from the egg (ovulation).

The environment of the ovary during this time is crucial. Proper nutrients and adequate blood flow to the reproductive system will enrich the environment in which the follicle is maturing and

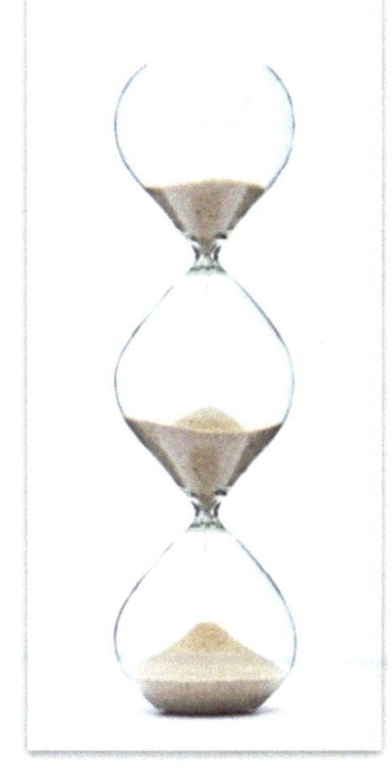

developing with the end result being better egg quality in the egg that is released 100 days later. So whatever you're doing now to improve your health will have a positive effect on the egg that is ovulated 100 days from now.

Fortunately, there are self-treatment options to enhance fertility and egg quality for natural fertility or in those 100 days prior to an IVF cycle.

Chapter

6

CHAPTER SIX: SECRET NO.3 - A WARM UTERUS

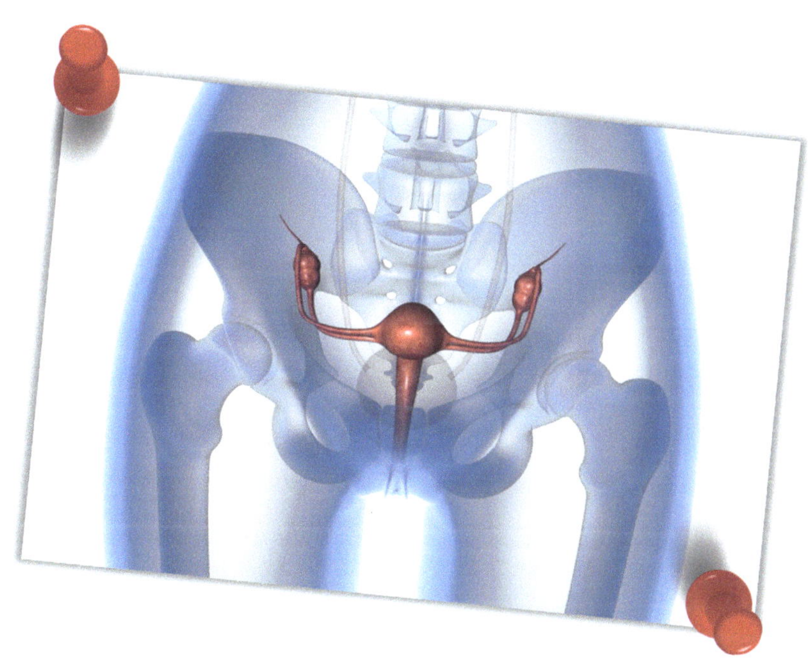

A warm uterus? I know this may sound foreign to you.

Dr. Jane Lyttleton, author of *Treatment of Infertility with Chinese Medicine* tells us that in Traditional Chinese Medicine "the warmth of the uterus refers to its metabolic activity, actively manufacturing the secreting nutrients and maintaining a highly nurturing home for a fetus".

As outlined earlier, Chinese medicine is always aiming to balance yin and yang. In the case of the opposite of a warm uterus, a cold uterus, the yang (warming) energy is inadequate causing the yin (cooling) energy to be in excess. A cold uterus is a very common gynecological pattern in Chinese medicine.

Yang energy is the catalyst for the body's physiological processes like the crucial reproductive processes of ovulation and proper implantation.

Maintaining a proper body temperature is always key when supporting optimal health and fertility.

When the uterus is cold, there is a lack of proper movement of blood. Cold has the property of constricting and blocking movement. This blocks proper blood flow.

A cold uterus hasn't responded well to the warming hormone progesterone. In Chinese medicine, estrogen is considered a more cooling hormone and progesterone is more warming.

A cold uterus is not an inviting, warm and hospitable environment for the growing fetus.

In the luteal phase, the second half of your cycle, the body temperature does go up in response to the warming hormone progesterone released by the corpus luteum. The reason for this is to be able to support embryo implantation.

Many women with recurrent miscarriages or unexplained infertility do have an underlying kidney yang deficiency. Kidney yang deficiency is connected to low progesterone and a lack of warmth in the body. Many women with kidney yang deficiency identify with having a luteal phase defect.

Signs and symptoms of a cold uterus:

Cold in the uterus consists of kidney yang deficiency signs plus blood stagnation signs.

- Difficulty getting pregnant is the first and most obvious sign
- Clots in the menstrual blood
- Dark blood (normal menstrual blood should be fresh red similar to the color of your blood when you cut yourself
- Delayed menstrual cycles meaning longer than 32 days (more like 35 days or longer)
- Severe menstrual cramps that get better with warmth
- Lower back pain
- Low sex drive
- Cold hands and especially cold feet
- Lower abdomen feels cooler to touch than the rest of your body (this is a big indication)
- Lower basal body temperature (BBT)

A cold uterus stems from the lack of kidney yang. Remember that yang is warmth. Lack of yang means there is not enough yang to push and move the blood which causes blood to stagnate or get blocked. An embryo can't implant and thrive in a cold stagnant uterus. Instead it needs warmth and a nutrient-rich blood supply.

How do we warm up the uterus?

Make sure that progesterone is at sufficient levels. This allows the uterus to secrete sufficient nutrients which creates a very nurturing environment for the embryo to implant in.

Unfortunately, in our society we eat way too many cold foods. Cold smoothies, big salads, sushi, ice cream, yogurt and the list goes on and on. We also drink too much cold iced beverages. Giving up some of the cold foods and incorporating more warming foods and drinks can actually be one of the most simple and yet most powerful changes you can make to support fertility.

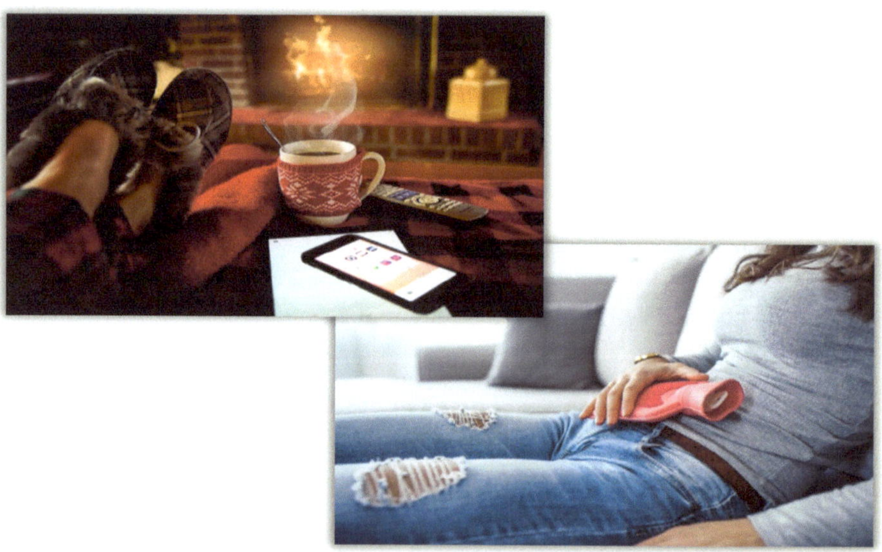

Some examples of other things I recommend are to wear socks and slippers and not walk barefoot on cold floors. The channels on the feet connect up into the uterus so it's essential to keep these meridians warm and not allow cold to enter the uterus.

Warm foot baths and heating pads over the lower abdomen are very helpful to warm the uterus too. Just note that heating pads should only be used before the embryo transfer if you're doing IVF and only in the first half of your menstrual cycle if trying naturally.

In my online program IVF With Confidence, I teach my patients many helpful tips, and the do's and don'ts to warm the uterus and supercharge an IVF cycle.

Chapter

7

CHAPTER SEVEN: SECRET NO.4 - CALM STRESS AND ANXIETY

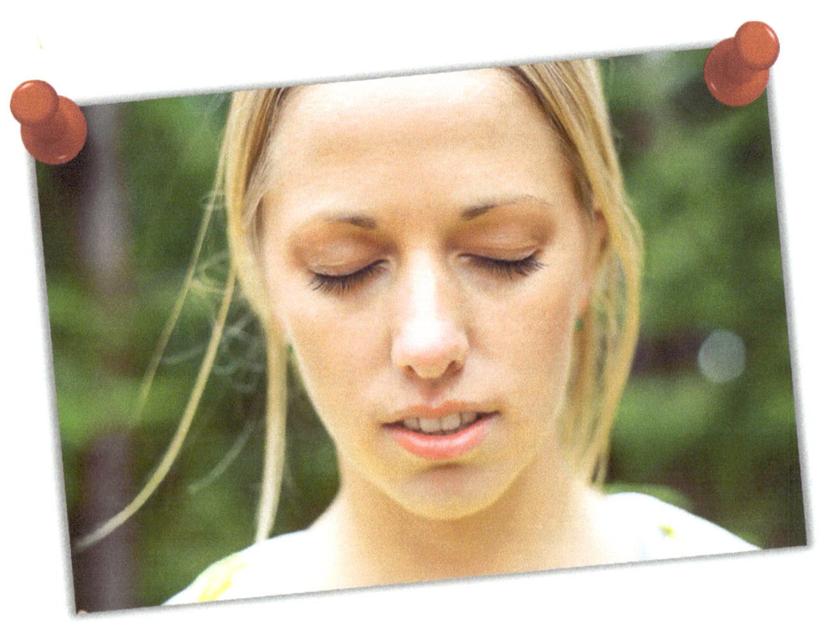

This can be one of the toughest aspects of the fertility process as the fertility journey can be one of the most stressful challenges couples go through. It involves a lot of patience, faith, heartbreak and dedication.

Especially when starting the IVF process, there comes a whole new set of pressures like numerous fertility appointments, invasive procedures, drug side effects and the financial burden.

Stress shows up as different physical symptoms and it varies among individuals. It could include insomnia, feeling restless, anxious or agitated, chest tightness and headaches to name a few.

Stress can compromise the immune system causing frequent colds and flus. It can also compromise hormone balance.

It probably comes as no surprise when you hear that stress doesn't do any good for your fertility and the success of your IVF cycle. Let's find out why.

STRESS CAN BLOCK FERTILITY

When we are stressed, our sympathetic nervous system is responding to stressors or threats and secretes the stress hormone cortisol.

Blood is diverted away from the reproductive system, digestive system and endocrine systems.

- the uterus and ovaries are deprived of nourishment
- the stomach may become prone to ulcers or other digestive problems
- blood may over-nourish some parts of the endocrine system while under-nourishing other parts causing hormonal imbalances and irregular menstrual cycles

A study of women undergoing IVF showed that those who had measurable lower levels of physiological stress had higher chances of pregnancy with IVF.

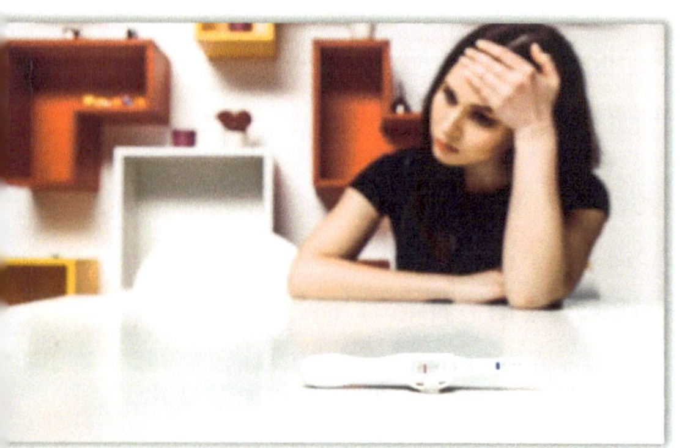

In regards to fertility, stress can cause ovulatory irregularities, absence of ovulation and abnormal sperm development.

Emotional stress can negatively affect the function of the hypothalamus which is the master control gland in the brain. The hypothalamus controls the endocrine (hormonal) system. When the hypothalamus is affected by emotional stress, this then affects the pituitary gland which can delay or switch off ovulation.

Stress causes blockage

In Chinese medicine, we call this Qi and blood stagnation. As you read in previous chapters, lack of blood flow can be detrimental to optimal fertility in the way of:

- follicular development in the ovaries
- poor egg quality
- irregular menstrual rhythm/cycle
- unfavorable uterus for implantation (meaning a thin uterine lining)
- and much more…

Liver Qi stagnation

In Chinese medicine, stress affects the liver organ system causing Liver Qi stagnation. You can picture Liver Qi stagnation as being wound up, tight, in pain, sighing a lot, feeling frustrated or angry. The most evident thing that can create Liver Qi stagnation is unfulfilled desires. These unfulfilled desires are quite apparent in women struggling with fertility and/or undergoing IVF. The strong desire to have your baby but not yet achieving that dream is disheartening to say the least.

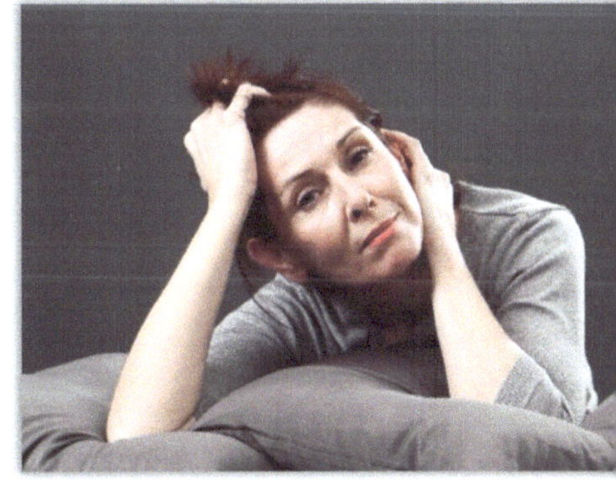

In my clinical practice, I see that most people have some degree of Liver Qi stagnation. In Chinese medicine, it is said "in adults blame the liver". The reason for this is that most (if not all) adults have some degree of unfulfilled desires. Children, on the other hand, don't have as much liver Qi stagnation because they tend to live in the moment.

The Liver channel pathway

The liver channel runs through the sides of the pelvic cavity, through the ovaries. If there is obstruction in the free flow of Qi and blood through this important channel, it can affect the function of the ovaries.

WHAT DOES LIVER QI STAGNATION LEAD TO?

Premenstrual Phase

The effects of liver Qi stagnation can be more obvious in the premenstrual phase because it is the Liver Qi that is responsible for moving the blood to begin menstruation. Premenstrual tension, breast fullness & soreness, irritability, depression and bloating can occur.

Liver Qi stagnation leads to blood deficiency

Blood deficiency is of paramount importance when it comes to gynecology and fertility. The liver stores the blood and provides

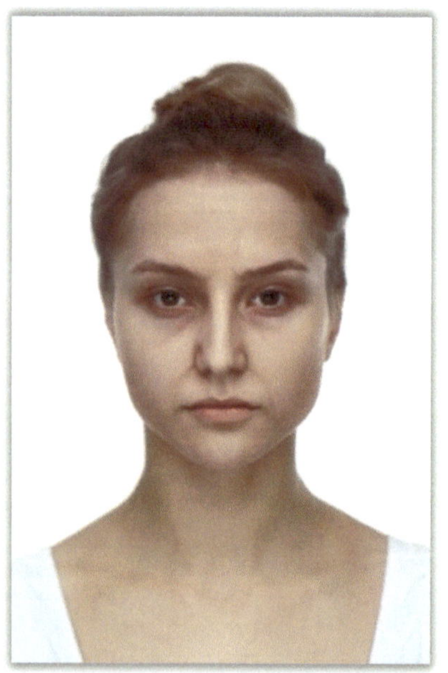

blood to the uterus. Women can be very prone to having deficiency of blood due to losing blood every month with their menstrual periods. Overwork, emotional stress and poor diet also have an important role to play in cases of blood deficiency.

Some signs of blood deficiency are light period flow, delayed menstrual cycle longer than 35 days, or no periods. Dry hair, dry skin, pale complexion and dizziness are also some common symptoms.3

Liver Qi stagnation leads to Spleen weakness

Have you ever been really anxious or nervous and as a result you had to run to the bathroom with diarrhea? Have you ever felt nauseated due to stress? These are some examples of Liver Qi stagnation causing spleen, or digestive, weakness. Remember that the spleen is in charge of digestion in Chinese medicine.

The spleen takes the nutrients and transforms it into Qi and blood. If the spleen becomes weak we will end up with Qi and blood deficiency and an undernourished reproductive system.

Liver Qi stagnation leads to heat

Over time, if liver Qi stagnation isn't resolved, it can lead to heat and inflammation in the body.

Put self-care and relaxation at the forefront before and during your IVF cycle. I know that while that may be easier said than done, my hope is that you can find ways to calm your mind and ease your heart for the sake of your fertility and IVF cycle. With my own patients, I show them self-acupressure techniques to do just this thru my program "IVF With Confidence".

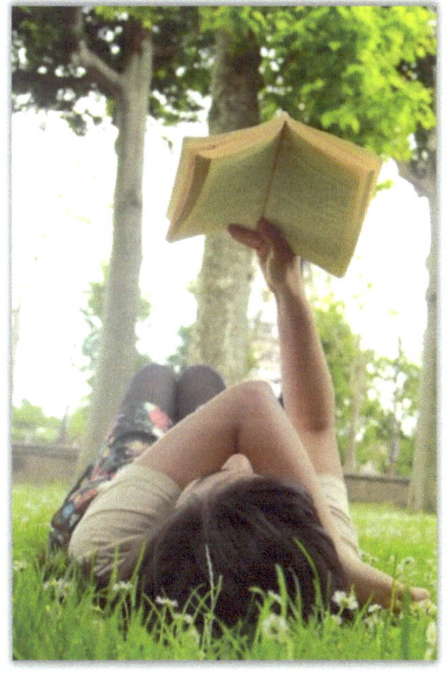

I also recommend simple meditation, regular acupuncture visits, moderate exercise like walking and being out in nature. I also highly recommend taking the time to do things that bring you joy. Perhaps chatting with a friend, watching a feel-good movie, reading your favorite book or whatever feels good for you.

Research Studies

There have been plenty of studies on acupuncture and IVF and the studies continue to evolve. These numerous research studies are generally outside the scope of this book.

2012 Meta-Analysis Research on IVF and acupuncture

A 2012 meta-analysis showed that acupuncture given with IVF cycles increases clinical pregnancy rates and live birth rates. Even more significant is when acupuncture is given at the time of ovarian stimulation and also at time of embryo transfer. This showed better results than acupuncture only at the time of the embryo transfer.

https://www.ncbi.nlm.nih.gov/pubmed/22243605

Colour-Doppler Study: This research showed that follicular development is directly correlated with blood supply. Greater quality blood supply to the follicles during ovarian stimulation has been associated with a greater likelihood of recovering a mature egg, higher grade embryos and better pregnancy outcomes. Poor blood supply can cause a longer stimulation phase and fewer eggs being recruited.

Closing Remarks

The purpose of writing this guide was to give you some insight into the unique perspectives of Chinese medicine when it comes to fertility and the IVF process. I hope it has shed some light on what Chinese medicine techniques can offer.

It should also be mentioned that the self-treatment tools and techniques that can be used to enhance the success of your IVF Cycle are well beyond the scope of this guide. However, you should know that you are only at the beginning of your journey and I encourage you to explore all your options, for example, taking an online self-treatment course.

My patients have seen great success with IVF With Confidence, a pre-recorded online course that teaches exact techniques, tools and practical tips to optimize your fertility at each stage of the IVF process, all performed from the comfort of your own home.

If you'd like more information, I am here to support you in your journey. My website has a wealth of free health resources that you may access to take greater control of your health: chinesemedicineclinic.com.

If you found this guide helpful and informative, please

encourage others who are dealing with fertility issues to read it.

My objective for you is that you gain more hope, confidence and peace of mind when embarking on your IVF journey and that you will utilize the wisdom of Chinese medicine in your path to better fertility and overall health.

With love and support,

Dr. Maryam

About Dr. Maryam

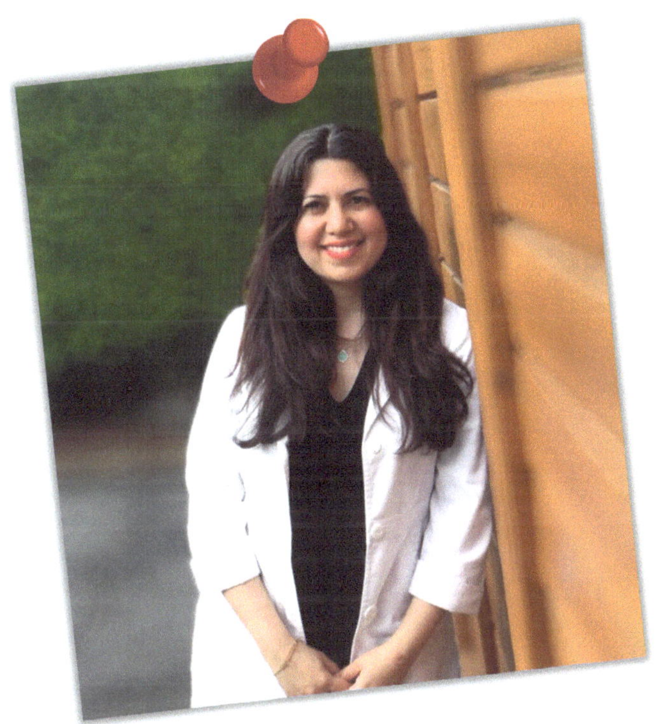

I started my Chinese medical education back in 1998. Being a natural holistic health advocate since a very young age, under the influence of my grandmother, studying Chinese medicine felt very appropriate. My grandmother was a sweet woman with a huge heart. Although she was illiterate as a result of her circumstances growing up, coming from a poor family in Iran, she was the wisest person I've known. She was also a natural healer. Whenever my sibling and I had tummy aches or colds and flus, she treated us quickly and effectively and never had to resort to pharmaceutical medications. I believe this is why natural remedies always felt right and I will forever rely and be a big believer in them.

I studied Chinese medicine at the International College of Traditional Chinese Medicine in Vancouver, BC Canada after studying general sciences at the University of British Columbia (UBC).

At the International College of Traditional Chinese Medicine (ICTCM) of Vancouver, I studied under prominent Chinese medicine doctors who had decades of knowledge and experience practicing in China. I was also privileged to go to China in my last year of school for an internship where I treated dozens of patients a day in many different departments of the hospitals including obstetrics and gynecology.

After having two children of my own, I knew that the area of women's health, fertility and pregnancy was an area I wanted to focus in my clinical practice.

I continue to strive to make sure my patients are heard, understood, and genuinely cared for and I treat my patients with compassion and a high level of knowledge and experience. Recently, I have also created a number of online self-treatment courses to help empower and educate people everywhere to improve their fertility and overall health from the comfort of their home and at their own pace using the practical tools based in Chinese medicine. I encourage you to learn more by visiting my website at chinesemedicineclinic.com.

Coupon

I believe that a woman's journey to better health and a more successful IVF cycle should be a right and not a privilege. Your decision to purchase this guide was the first step along this path.

E-COUPON [$100]

IVF WITH CONFIDENCE
ONLINE SELF-TREATMENT COURSE

As a measure of my gratitude to you for purchasing this guide, I am gifting you a one-time special **e-coupon in the amount of $100 (CAD)** that can be applied against the cost of enrolling in my comprehensive online self-treatment course "IVF With Confidence".

The course includes approximately 30 pre-recorded video lessons and how-to tutorials, as well as printable PDF guides and cheats sheets. This course essentially picks up where this guide leaves off.

Learn more by visiting the course page of my website: chinesemedicineclinic.com.

If you decide that this is right for you, please email me at drmahanian@chinesemedicineclinic.com to receive a one-time coupon code.

Follow me

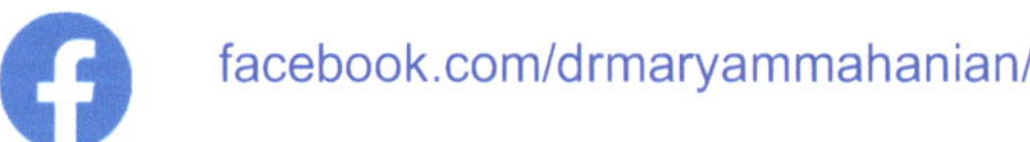
facebook.com/drmaryammahanian/

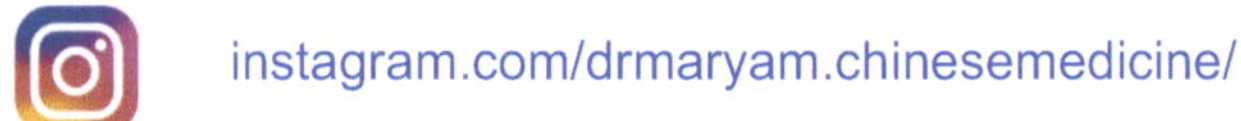
instagram.com/drmaryam.chinesemedicine/

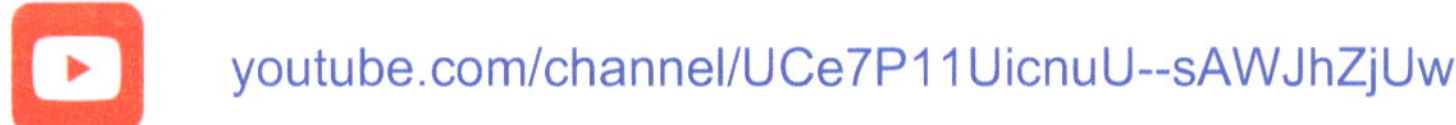
youtube.com/channel/UCe7P11UicnuU--sAWJhZjUw

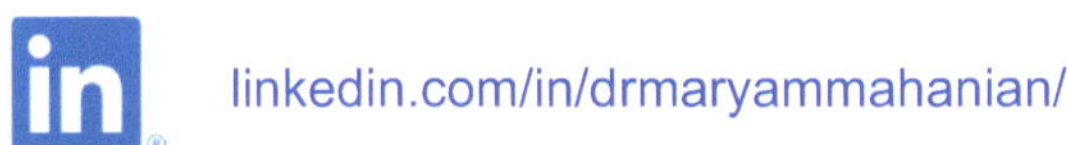
linkedin.com/in/drmaryammahanian/

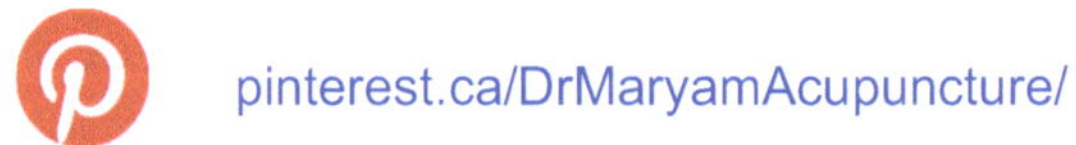
pinterest.ca/DrMaryamAcupuncture/

Dr. Maryam Mahanian *is a doctor of Chinese medicine and registered acupuncturist. She has been successfully treating patients since 2002 using acupuncture and other natural medical techniques based on the science and wisdom of an age-old medical practice known as Traditional Chinese Medicine (TCM). Dr. Maryam has appeared on TV and in mainstream magazine publications and public webinars. She built her medical career based on two decades of hands on experience.*